Nurses
Reflection Diary
Revalidation ✓

Version 2

Jane Coombs

Dedication

For all nurses and midwives everywhere.
The doers and thinkers

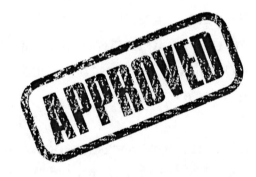

How to Use this Book

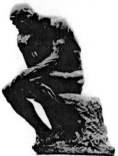

In order to maintain registration with the Nursing Midwifery Council (NMC) in the UK, nurses and midwives must keep up to date with current evidence based or best practice, and change with the times. Continuing professional development or CPD, is an integral part of maintaining standards throughout the nursing profession.

One part of demonstrating CPD is to reflect on incidents, learning or feedback and consider if you need to change your practice – could you have done things better? Do you have the right tools and resources to do your job?

Formal reflection gives nurses and midwives time to stop and think about their own practice and identify personal issues, such as how you communicate, training requirements, and so on. Reflection can also highlight blocks in your workplace systems, unworkable practices that need reviewing or the need for more resources where you work.

The incidents or feedback you chose for reflection are for you to choose but must be linked to the code of practice for nurses. Found on line at http://www.nmc.org.uk/standards/code/

The most common type of reflection is usually after a situation which hasn't turned out as planned, or when negative feedback is given. However, you should also consider improving good situations and reflecting on how you can have done things even better.

Included in this work book is a reflective model (Gibbs) which I have adapted to fit the six stage model. I have also added an example of a reflective piece showing how each element fits into the cycle of reflection, action and improvement.

You will find an image of the model within each reflective record for easy reference.

I have also included a summary of the NMC code of practice so that you can easily link your incident to the appropriate part of the code, although you may need to go to the NMC website for in depth information if you can't decide.

This book is a way of recording your reflective pieces over the years. You can chose any or all of the reflections for revalidation purposes.

At the back of the book you will find forms for your professional supervisor to complete, which you can photocopy, photograph or scan and put in your personal professional portfolio for review by confirmer, prior to revalidation with the NMC.

For more in depth information about revalidation go to Nursing Midwifery Council website at www.nmc.org.uk

For more information about me and my practice, why not visit my website at www.workingwellsolutions.com

"I cannot teach anybody anything.

I can only make them think"

Socrates

NMC Code Links

Link each reflection to one of the tenets of the Code:

Prioritise People

1 Treat people as individuals and uphold their dignity
2 Listen to people and respond to their preferences and concerns
3 Make sure that people's physical, social and psychological needs are assessed and responded to
4 Act in the best interests of people at all times
5 Respect people's right to privacy and confidentiality

Practise Effectively

6 Always practise in line with the best available evidence
7 Communicate clearly
8 Work cooperatively
9 Share your skills, knowledge and experience for the benefit of people receiving care and your colleagues
10 Keep clear and accurate records relevant to your practice
11 Be accountable for your decisions to delegate tasks and duties to other people
12 Have in place an indemnity arrangement which provides appropriate cover for any practice you take on as a nurse or midwife in the United Kingdom

Preserve Safety

13 Recognise and work within the limits of your competence

14 Be open and candid with all service users about all aspects of care and treatment, including when any mistakes or harm have taken place

15 Always offer help if an emergency arises in your practice setting or anywhere else

16 Act without delay if you believe that there is a risk to patient safety or public protection

17 Raise concerns immediately if you believe a person is vulnerable or at risk and needs extra support and protection

18 Advise on, prescribe, supply, dispense or administer medicines within the limits of your training and competence, the law, our guidance and other relevant policies, guidance and regulations

19 Be aware of, and reduce as far as possible, any potential for harm associated with your practice

Promote Professionalism and Trust

20 Uphold the reputation of your profession at all times

21 Uphold your position as a registered nurse or midwife

22 Fulfil all registration requirements

23 Cooperate with all investigations and audits

24 Respond to any complaints made against you professionally

25 Provide leadership to make sure people's wellbeing is protected and to improve their experiences of the healthcare system

Full details available on line at:
http://www.nmc.org.uk/standards/code/read-the-code-online/

Adapted Gibbs Reflection Model

A Framework for Reflection

Gibbs (1998) developed a reflective cycle structure which I have adapted for reflecting on a nursing experience or situation.

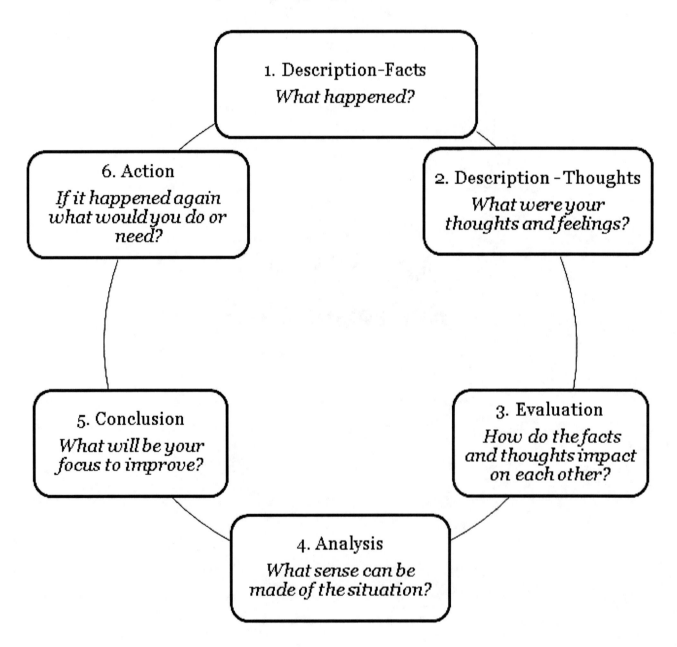

1. Description-Facts
What happened?

2. Description - Thoughts
What were your thoughts and feelings?

3. Evaluation
How do the facts and thoughts impact on each other?

4. Analysis
What sense can be made of the situation?

5. Conclusion
What will be your focus to improve?

6. Action
If it happened again what would you do or need?

To see if Gibb's reflective cycle can help you reflect on aspects of your practice, recall a nursing situation that you were involved in that didn't turn out as you expected or go to plan.

Stage 1 - Description (Pure Facts)

- What are the brief facts of the situation?
- What occurred? Who was involved?
- What did you do? What did others do?

Stage 2 - Description (Thoughts)

- How were you feeling at the time?
- Were there influences affecting others actions/behaviour?
- Were there any known or perceived difficulties with the activity, timing, location, information or resources etc?

Stage 3 - Evaluation

- What was good and bad about the experience
- How might the facts and feelings (from stage 1 and 2 above) have affected your actions/behaviour
- What other circumstances may have affected your actions or thoughts?
- How issues might influence the activity or practice related feedback?

Stage 4 - Analysis

- Why you picked this incident to reflect on?
- What sense can you make of it? Does it make sense given the preceding 3 stages
- What is the main area of concern or focus for the future?

Stage 5 - Conclusions

- What have you discovered?
- What have you learned from this incident and circumstances?
- What questions remain?

Stage 6 - Action

- What will I do differently from now on or the next time this arises?
- What resources/help will I need?

Reference

Gibbs, (1988) Learning by Doing: A Guide to Teaching and Learning Methods Further Education Unit, Oxford Brookes University, Oxford.

Example Reflection

Using the Adapted Gibbs Reflection Model

Stage 1 - Description - Facts

I was a 3rd year student nurse on night duty. A doctor asked me to give a patient 0.1 mgs of Digoxin to a patient with congestive cardiac failure. I had never given this dose before and measured 4 tabs from the 0.25 mgs bottle. I checked the script and the tabs with both the doctor and my junior nurse before giving the tablets. Who all agreed with my actions. Mrs X was pretty unwell and we kept her on hourly observations throughout the night. At about 2 am I suddenly realised that I had given 10 times the amount stated on the Doctors script.

I called the night sister who agreed that I had. We filled in an incident form, informed the doctor and Mrs x's relatives of what had happened and I had to see the hospital matron in the morning. Mrs x did not seem to suffer any ill effects from the Digoxin. And went on to make a full recovery.

Stage 2 – Description - (Thoughts)

I had been on nights for a long stretch. It was a very busy ward with only two night staff for 22 patients. Mrs X was very ill and needed constant monitoring. I had only ever seen .25mgs of Digoxin and did not know there was a paediatric blue table of 0.1 mgs made. I was very reluctant to give such a big dose which is why I checked the four tablets of .25 with the doctor who looked at the tablets and said OK. I was nervous about the dosage being so high.
The doctor too was under tremendous strain, his bleeper kept going off and he was rushing about all over the place. I had never met him before. He had recently come from a paediatric ward.

Stage 3 - Evaluation

Nobody ever blamed me for the incident, neither did they reassure me. Mrs X went on to make a full recovery and the relatives were very understanding about the situation. Matron was kind to me and impressed that I had actually owned up to the error – nobody would have ever known, she said.
I felt absolutely terrified about the error though and watched Mrs X all night for signs of overdose. I didn't sleep all the next day and returned to my next night shift to find Mrs X much better.

Stage 4 - Analysis

This incident really frightened me because I had done everything right - I had checked the dosage with both the Doctor and the junior nurse. I had not known that you could get a 0.1 mg of Digoxin or that it was blue. I have no idea what prompted me to think about the overdose later on that night except that I had been very reluctant to give it. The Doctor agreed I had shown him 4 white tablets

"I thought you knew what you were doing" He'd said

Which isn't any sort of answer really. Yet he didn't get in any kind of trouble at all for overseeing and agreeing my mistake.

I believe that this incident was due to a series of incidents linked to overwork, tiredness and misunderstandings.

Stage 5 - Conclusions

I was so relieved that Mrs X survived the overdose and that the relatives were understanding but, if she had had a serious reaction or even died, I'm not sure I could have carried on nursing.

Stage 6 - Action

I have learnt to be more careful with drugs and to really understand the dosage. If necessary now I will look up the drug in the reference books before I give them because at the end of the day, it will be my responsibility if I do it wrong.

I will always be ultra-careful with new drug scripts in the future and if I am nervous, then to go with my gut feel and check and check again. Although, as I said to Matron, at the time I'd felt as if I done as much as I could have done. Also, if nurses in my team are involved in incidents where they have made a clinical mistake, I am always on hand to offer support and an opportunity to talk to me.

I link this reflection to "Preserving Safety" (14) from the NMC Code for Nurses

The Diary

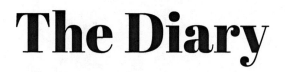

Name_____

NMC Pin Number_____   Revalidation Due_____

Incident Date_____   Date of Reflection_____

Nature of the CPD activity/practice related feedback

Description Stage 1: Facts

_____
_____
_____
_____
_____
_____
_____
_____
_____

Description Stage 2: Feelings

_____
_____
_____
_____
_____
_____
_____
_____
_____
_____
_____

A Framework for Reflection

Gibbs (1998) developed a reflective cycle structure which I have adapted for reflecting on a nursing experience or situation.

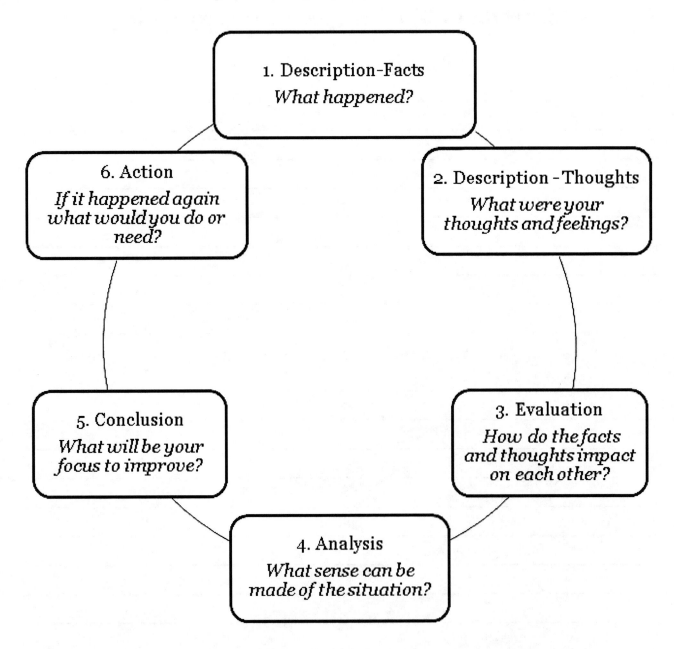

Stage 3: Evaluation and Stage 4: Analysis

_____

_____

_____

_____

_____

_____

_____

_____

_____

_____

_____

_____

_____

_____

_____

_____

_____

Stage 5: Conclusions

_____

_____

_____

_____

_____

_____

_____

_____

_____

_____

_____

_____

_____

Relevance to the NMC Code of Practice

Prioritise People ☐

Practice Effectively ☐

Preserve Safety ☐

Promote Professionalism and Trust ☐

Stage 6: Action Plan For Improvement

_____
_____
_____
_____
_____
_____
_____
_____
_____

Notes and Links to Evidence

_____
_____
_____
_____
_____

Discussed with Professional Assessor ☐

Signature_____**Date Completed**_____

Name_____

NMC Pin Number_____ **Revalidation Due**_____

Incident Date_____ **Date of Reflection**_____

Nature of the CPD activity/practice related feedback

Description Stage 1: Facts

_____
_____
_____
_____
_____
_____
_____
_____
_____

Description Stage 2: Feelings

_____
_____
_____
_____
_____
_____
_____
_____
_____
_____

A Framework for Reflection

Gibbs (1998) developed a reflective cycle structure which I have adapted for reflecting on a nursing experience or situation.

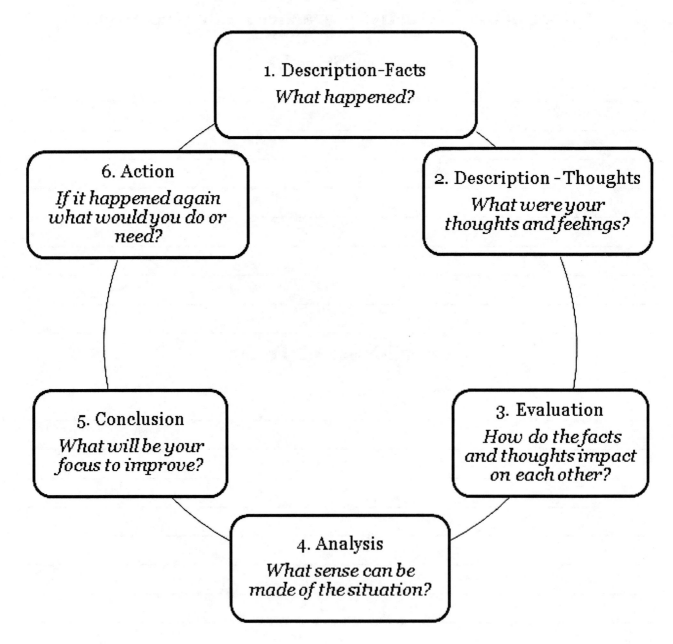

1. Description-Facts
What happened?

2. Description -Thoughts
What were your thoughts and feelings?

3. Evaluation
How do the facts and thoughts impact on each other?

4. Analysis
What sense can be made of the situation?

5. Conclusion
What will be your focus to improve?

6. Action
If it happened again what would you do or need?

Stage 3: Evaluation and Stage 4: Analysis

_____
_____
_____
_____
_____
_____
_____
_____
_____
_____
_____
_____
_____
_____
_____
_____

Stage 5: Conclusions

_____
_____
_____
_____
_____
_____
_____
_____
_____
_____
_____
_____
_____
_____

Relevance to the NMC Code of Practice

Prioritise People ☐   **Practice Effectively** ☐

Preserve Safety ☐   **Promote Professionalism and Trust** ☐

Stage 6: Action Plan For Improvement

_____
_____
_____
_____
_____
_____
_____
_____
_____
_____

Notes and Links to Evidence

_____
_____
_____
_____
_____

Discussed with Professional Assessor ☐

Signature_____**Date Completed**_____

Name_____

NMC Pin Number_____   **Revalidation Due**_____

Incident Date_____   **Date of Reflection**_____

Nature of the CPD activity/practice related feedback

Description Stage 1: Facts

_____

_____

_____

_____

_____

_____

_____

_____

_____

Description Stage 2: Feelings

_____

_____

_____

_____

_____

_____

_____

_____

_____

_____

_____

A Framework for Reflection

Gibbs (1998) developed a reflective cycle structure which I have adapted for reflecting on a nursing experience or situation.

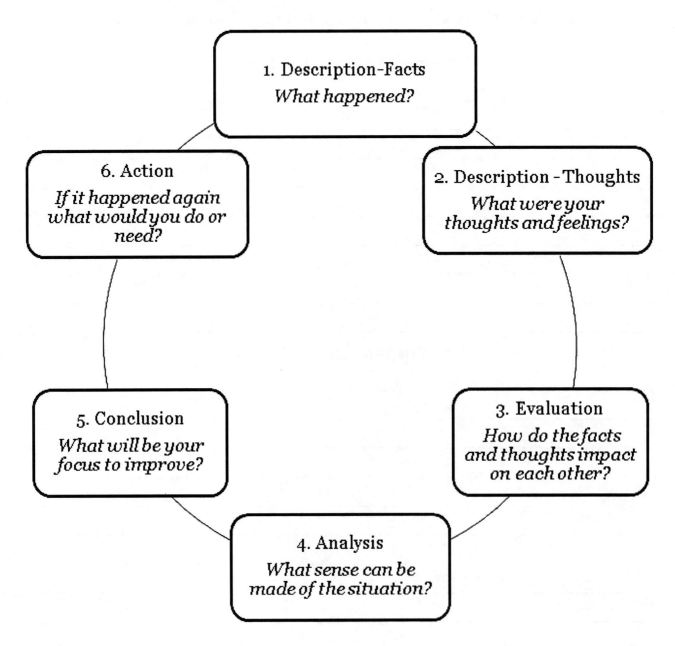

Stage 3: Evaluation and Stage 4: Analysis

_____
_____
_____
_____
_____
_____
_____
_____
_____
_____
_____
_____
_____
_____
_____
_____

Stage 5: Conclusions

_____
_____
_____
_____
_____
_____
_____
_____
_____
_____
_____
_____
_____
_____

Relevance to the NMC Code of Practice

Prioritise People ☐   **Practice Effectively** ☐

Preserve Safety ☐   **Promote Professionalism and Trust** ☐

Stage 6: Action Plan For Improvement

_____
_____
_____
_____
_____
_____
_____
_____
_____
_____

Notes and Links to Evidence

_____
_____
_____
_____
_____

Discussed with Professional Assessor ☐

Signature_____**Date Completed**_____

Name_____

NMC Pin Number_____ **Revalidation Due**_____

Incident Date_____ **Date of Reflection**_____

Nature of the CPD activity/practice related feedback

Description Stage 1: Facts

_____
_____
_____
_____
_____
_____
_____
_____
_____

Description Stage 2: Feelings

_____
_____
_____
_____
_____
_____
_____
_____
_____
_____
_____

A Framework for Reflection

Gibbs (1998) developed a reflective cycle structure which I have adapted for reflecting on a nursing experience or situation.

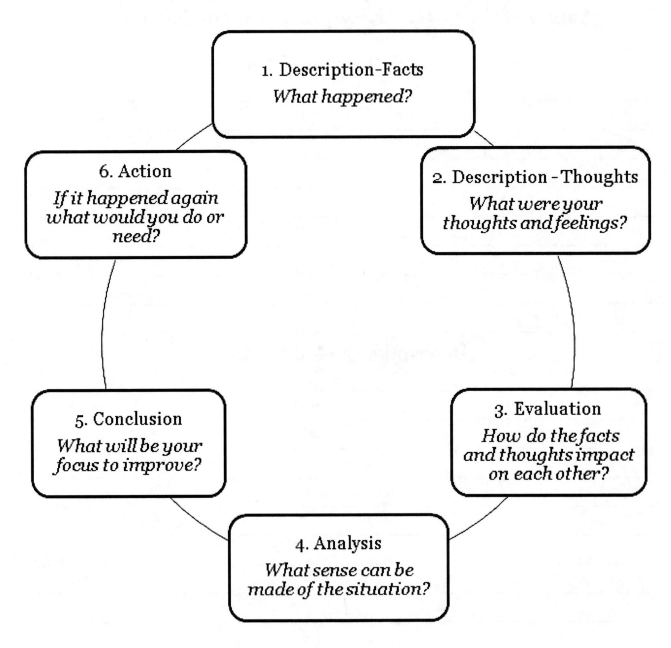

Stage 3: Evaluation and Stage 4: Analysis

_____

_____

_____

_____

_____

_____

_____

_____

_____

_____

_____

_____

_____

_____

Stage 5: Conclusions

_____

_____

_____

_____

_____

_____

_____

_____

_____

_____

_____

_____

Relevance to the NMC Code of Practice

Prioritise People ☐   **Practice Effectively** ☐

Preserve Safety ☐   **Promote Professionalism and Trust** ☐

Stage 6: Action Plan For Improvement

_____
_____
_____
_____
_____
_____
_____
_____
_____
_____

Notes and Links to Evidence

_____
_____
_____
_____
_____

Discussed with Professional Assessor ☐

Signature_____**Date Completed**_____

Name_____

NMC Pin Number_____   Revalidation Due_____

Incident Date_____   Date of Reflection_____

Nature of the CPD activity/practice related feedback

Description Stage 1: Facts

_____
_____
_____
_____
_____
_____
_____
_____
_____

Description Stage 2: Feelings

_____
_____
_____
_____
_____
_____
_____
_____
_____
_____
_____

A Framework for Reflection

Gibbs (1998) developed a reflective cycle structure which I have adapted for reflecting on a nursing experience or situation.

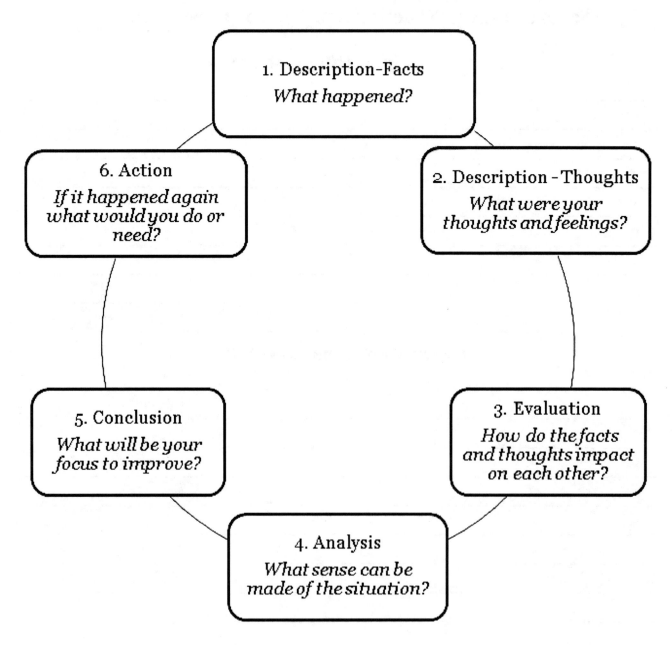

1. Description-Facts
What happened?

2. Description - Thoughts
What were your thoughts and feelings?

3. Evaluation
How do the facts and thoughts impact on each other?

4. Analysis
What sense can be made of the situation?

5. Conclusion
What will be your focus to improve?

6. Action
If it happened again what would you do or need?

Stage 3: Evaluation and Stage 4: Analysis

_____

_____

_____

_____

_____

_____

_____

_____

_____

_____

_____

_____

_____

_____

_____

Stage 5: Conclusions

_____

_____

_____

_____

_____

_____

_____

_____

_____

_____

_____

_____

_____

Relevance to the NMC Code of Practice

Prioritise People ☐   **Practice Effectively** ☐

Preserve Safety ☐   **Promote Professionalism and Trust** ☐

Stage 6: Action Plan For Improvement

_____
_____
_____
_____
_____
_____
_____
_____
_____
_____

Notes and Links to Evidence

_____
_____
_____
_____
_____

Discussed with Professional Assessor ☐

Signature_____**Date Completed**_____

Name_____

NMC Pin Number_____   **Revalidation Due**_____

Incident Date_____   **Date of Reflection**_____

Nature of the CPD activity/practice related feedback

Description Stage 1: Facts

_____
_____
_____
_____
_____
_____
_____
_____
_____
_____

Description Stage 2: Feelings

_____
_____
_____
_____
_____
_____
_____
_____
_____
_____

A Framework for Reflection

Gibbs (1998) developed a reflective cycle structure which I have adapted for reflecting on a nursing experience or situation.

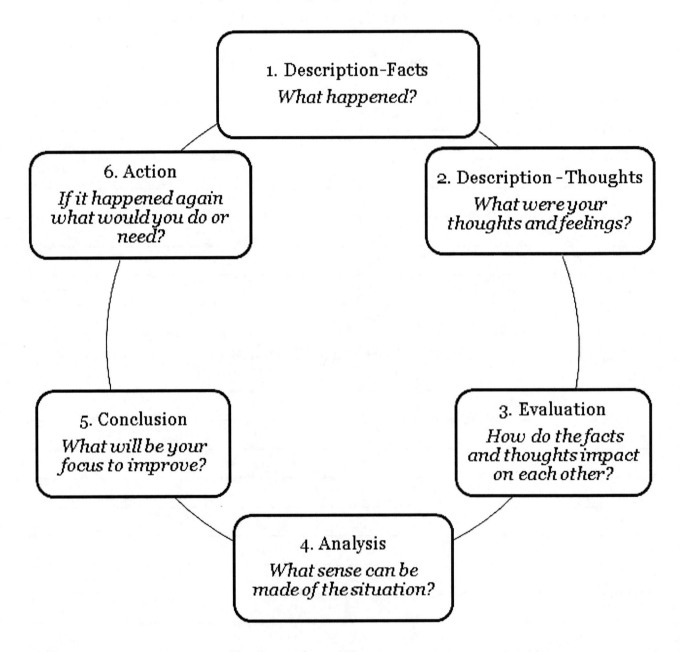

1. Description-Facts
What happened?

2. Description - Thoughts
What were your thoughts and feelings?

3. Evaluation
How do the facts and thoughts impact on each other?

4. Analysis
What sense can be made of the situation?

5. Conclusion
What will be your focus to improve?

6. Action
If it happened again what would you do or need?

Stage 3: Evaluation and Stage 4: Analysis

_____
_____
_____
_____
_____
_____
_____
_____
_____
_____
_____
_____
_____
_____
_____
_____
_____

Stage 5: Conclusions

_____
_____
_____
_____
_____
_____
_____
_____
_____
_____
_____
_____
_____

Relevance to the NMC Code of Practice

Prioritise People ☐

Practice Effectively ☐

Preserve Safety ☐

Promote Professionalism and Trust ☐

Stage 6: Action Plan For Improvement

_____
_____
_____
_____
_____
_____
_____
_____
_____

Notes and Links to Evidence

_____
_____
_____
_____
_____

Discussed with Professional Assessor ☐

Signature_____**Date Completed**_____

Name_____

NMC Pin Number_____   **Revalidation Due**_____

Incident Date_____   **Date of Reflection**_____

Nature of the CPD activity/practice related feedback

Description Stage 1: Facts

_____
_____
_____
_____
_____
_____
_____
_____
_____

Description Stage 2: Feelings

_____
_____
_____
_____
_____
_____
_____
_____
_____

A Framework for Reflection

Gibbs (1998) developed a reflective cycle structure which I have adapted for reflecting on a nursing experience or situation.

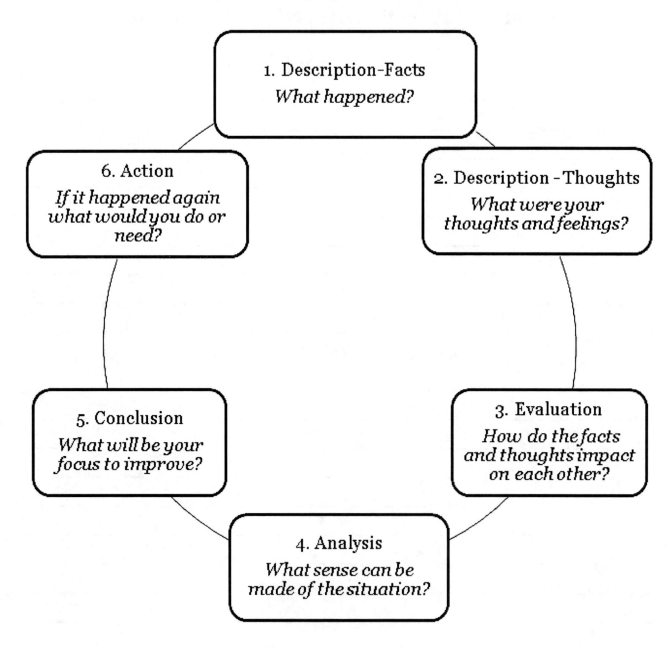

Stage 3: Evaluation and Stage 4: Analysis

_____
_____
_____
_____
_____
_____
_____
_____
_____
_____
_____
_____
_____
_____
_____
_____
_____

Stage 5: Conclusions

_____
_____
_____
_____
_____
_____
_____
_____
_____
_____
_____
_____
_____
_____

Relevance to the NMC Code of Practice

Prioritise People ☐   **Practice Effectively** ☐

Preserve Safety ☐   **Promote Professionalism and Trust** ☐

Stage 6: Action Plan For Improvement

_____

_____

_____

_____

_____

_____

_____

_____

_____

Notes and Links to Evidence

_____

_____

_____

_____

_____

Discussed with Professional Assessor ☐

Signature_____**Date Completed**_____

Name_____

NMC Pin Number_____   **Revalidation Due**_____

Incident Date_____   **Date of Reflection**_____

Nature of the CPD activity/practice related feedback

Description Stage 1: Facts

_____
_____
_____
_____
_____
_____
_____
_____
_____

Description Stage 2: Feelings

_____
_____
_____
_____
_____
_____
_____
_____
_____
_____
_____

A Framework for Reflection

Gibbs (1998) developed a reflective cycle structure which I have adapted for reflecting on a nursing experience or situation.

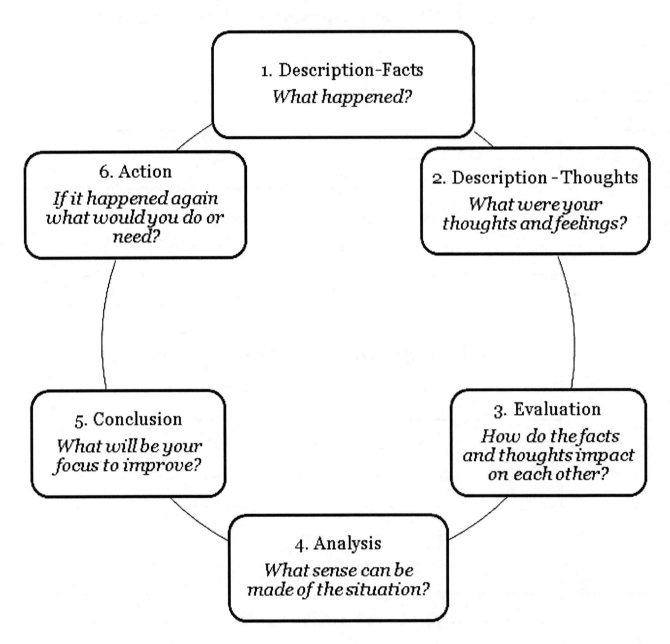

1. Description-Facts
What happened?

2. Description - Thoughts
What were your thoughts and feelings?

3. Evaluation
How do the facts and thoughts impact on each other?

4. Analysis
What sense can be made of the situation?

5. Conclusion
What will be your focus to improve?

6. Action
If it happened again what would you do or need?

Stage 3: Evaluation and Stage 4: Analysis

_____
_____
_____
_____
_____
_____
_____
_____
_____
_____
_____
_____
_____
_____
_____
_____
_____

Stage 5: Conclusions

_____
_____
_____
_____
_____
_____
_____
_____
_____
_____
_____
_____
_____
_____
_____

Relevance to the NMC Code of Practice

Prioritise People ☐   **Practice Effectively** ☐

Preserve Safety ☐   **Promote Professionalism and Trust** ☐

Stage 6: Action Plan For Improvement

_____

_____

_____

_____

_____

_____

_____

_____

_____

Notes and Links to Evidence

_____

_____

_____

_____

_____

Discussed with Professional Assessor ☐

Signature_____**Date Completed**_____

Name_____

NMC Pin Number_____   **Revalidation Due**_____

Incident Date_____   **Date of Reflection**_____

Nature of the CPD activity/practice related feedback

Description Stage 1: Facts

_____

_____

_____

_____

_____

_____

_____

_____

_____

Description Stage 2: Feelings

_____

_____

_____

_____

_____

_____

_____

_____

_____

_____

A Framework for Reflection

Gibbs (1998) developed a reflective cycle structure which I have adapted for reflecting on a nursing experience or situation.

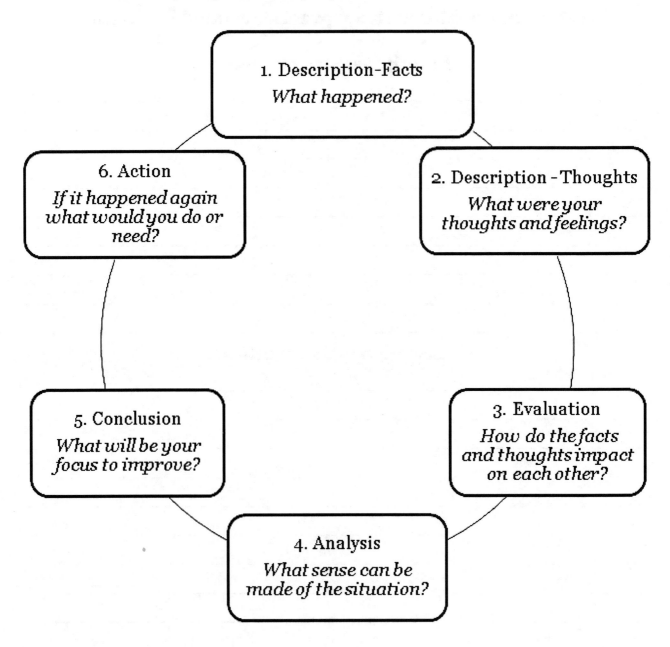

Stage 3: Evaluation and Stage 4: Analysis

_____
_____
_____
_____
_____
_____
_____
_____
_____
_____
_____
_____
_____
_____
_____
_____

Stage 5: Conclusions

_____
_____
_____
_____
_____
_____
_____
_____
_____
_____
_____
_____
_____
_____
_____

Relevance to the NMC Code of Practice

Prioritise People ☐   **Practice Effectively** ☐

Preserve Safety ☐   **Promote Professionalism and Trust** ☐

Stage 6: Action Plan For Improvement

_____

_____

_____

_____

_____

_____

_____

_____

_____

Notes and Links to Evidence

_____

_____

_____

_____

_____

Discussed with Professional Assessor ☐

Signature_____**Date Completed**_____

Name_____

NMC Pin Number_____   Revalidation Due_____

Incident Date_____   Date of Reflection_____

Nature of the CPD activity/practice related feedback

Description Stage 1: Facts

_____
_____
_____
_____
_____
_____
_____
_____
_____

Description Stage 2: Feelings

_____
_____
_____
_____
_____
_____
_____
_____
_____
_____

A Framework for Reflection

Gibbs (1998) developed a reflective cycle structure which I have adapted for reflecting on a nursing experience or situation.

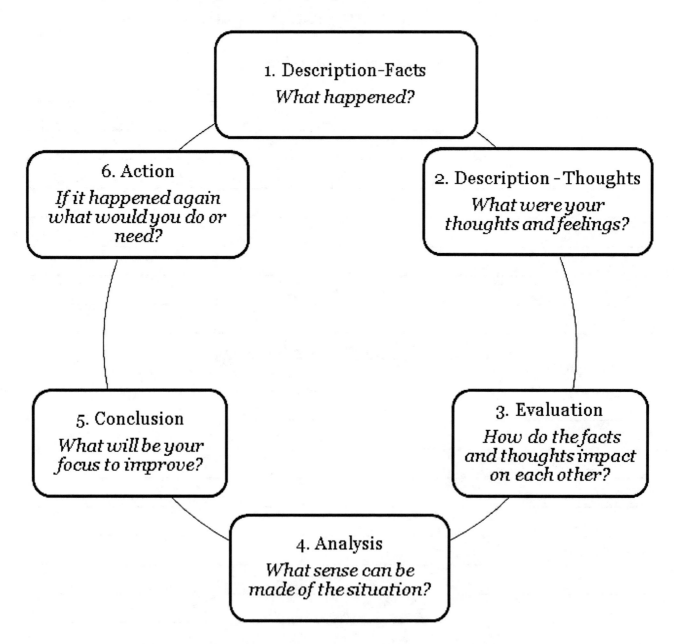

1. Description-Facts
What happened?

2. Description -Thoughts
What were your thoughts and feelings?

3. Evaluation
How do the facts and thoughts impact on each other?

4. Analysis
What sense can be made of the situation?

5. Conclusion
What will be your focus to improve?

6. Action
If it happened again what would you do or need?

Stage 3: Evaluation and Stage 4: Analysis

_____
_____
_____
_____
_____
_____
_____
_____
_____
_____
_____
_____
_____
_____

Stage 5: Conclusions

_____
_____
_____
_____
_____
_____
_____
_____
_____
_____
_____
_____
_____

Relevance to the NMC Code of Practice

Prioritise People ☐   **Practice Effectively** ☐

Preserve Safety ☐   **Promote Professionalism and Trust** ☐

Stage 6: Action Plan For Improvement

_____

_____

_____

_____

_____

_____

_____

_____

_____

_____

Notes and Links to Evidence

_____

_____

_____

_____

_____

Discussed with Professional Assessor ☐

Signature_____**Date Completed**_____

Name_____

NMC Pin Number_____   Revalidation Due_____

Incident Date_____   Date of Reflection_____

Nature of the CPD activity/practice related feedback

Description Stage 1: Facts

_____
_____
_____
_____
_____
_____
_____
_____
_____

Description Stage 2: Feelings

_____
_____
_____
_____
_____
_____
_____
_____
_____
_____

A Framework for Reflection

Gibbs (1998) developed a reflective cycle structure which I have adapted for reflecting on a nursing experience or situation.

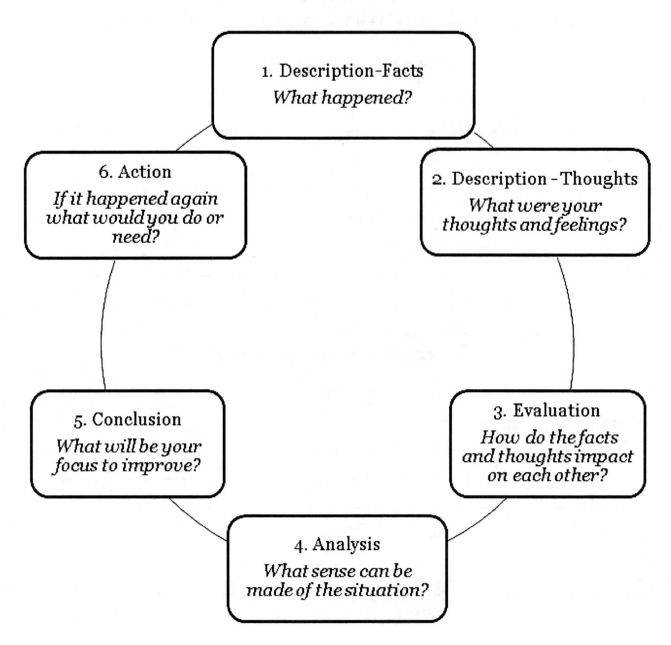

1. Description-Facts
What happened?

2. Description - Thoughts
What were your thoughts and feelings?

3. Evaluation
How do the facts and thoughts impact on each other?

4. Analysis
What sense can be made of the situation?

5. Conclusion
What will be your focus to improve?

6. Action
If it happened again what would you do or need?

Stage 3: Evaluation and Stage 4: Analysis

_____
_____
_____
_____
_____
_____
_____
_____
_____
_____
_____
_____
_____
_____
_____
_____

Stage 5: Conclusions

_____
_____
_____
_____
_____
_____
_____
_____
_____
_____
_____
_____
_____
_____

Relevance to the NMC Code of Practice

Prioritise People ☐   **Practice Effectively** ☐

Preserve Safety ☐   **Promote Professionalism and Trust** ☐

Stage 6: Action Plan For Improvement

_____
_____
_____
_____
_____
_____
_____
_____
_____
_____

Notes and Links to Evidence

_____
_____
_____
_____
_____

Discussed with Professional Assessor ☐

Signature_____**Date Completed**_____

Name_____

NMC Pin Number_____ **Revalidation Due**_____

Incident Date_____ **Date of Reflection**_____

Nature of the CPD activity/practice related feedback

Description Stage 1: Facts

_____
_____
_____
_____
_____
_____
_____
_____
_____

Description Stage 2: Feelings

_____
_____
_____
_____
_____
_____
_____
_____
_____
_____

A Framework for Reflection

Gibbs (1998) developed a reflective cycle structure which I have adapted for reflecting on a nursing experience or situation.

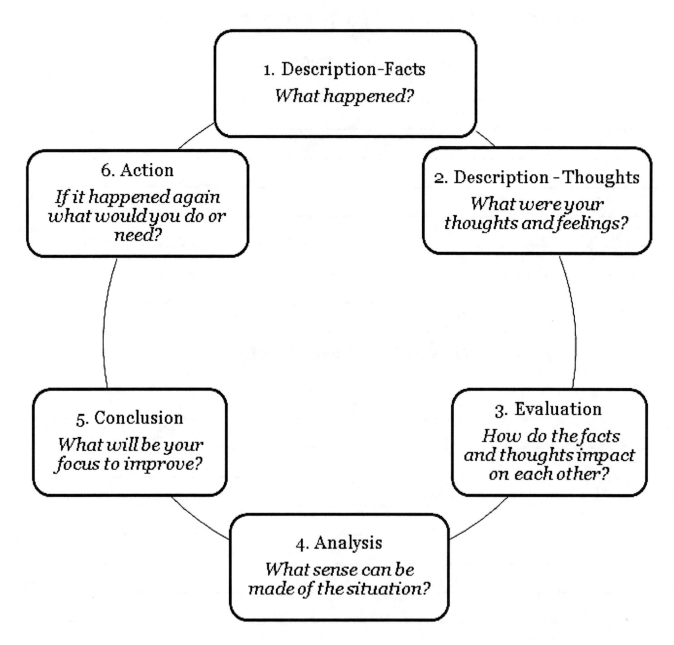

1. Description-Facts
What happened?

2. Description -Thoughts
What were your thoughts and feelings?

3. Evaluation
How do the facts and thoughts impact on each other?

4. Analysis
What sense can be made of the situation?

5. Conclusion
What will be your focus to improve?

6. Action
If it happened again what would you do or need?

Stage 3: Evaluation and Stage 4: Analysis

_____

_____

_____

_____

_____

_____

_____

_____

_____

_____

_____

_____

_____

_____

_____

_____

Stage 5: Conclusions

_____

_____

_____

_____

_____

_____

_____

_____

_____

_____

_____

_____

_____

Relevance to the NMC Code of Practice

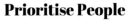

Prioritise People ☐   **Practice Effectively** ☐

Preserve Safety ☐   **Promote Professionalism and Trust** ☐

Stage 6: Action Plan For Improvement

_____
_____
_____
_____
_____
_____
_____
_____
_____

Notes and Links to Evidence

_____
_____
_____
_____
_____

Discussed with Professional Assessor ☐

Signature_____**Date Completed**_____

Name_____

NMC Pin Number_____   Revalidation Due_____

Incident Date_____   Date of Reflection_____

Nature of the CPD activity/practice related feedback

Description Stage 1: Facts

_____
_____
_____
_____
_____
_____
_____
_____
_____

Description Stage 2: Feelings

_____
_____
_____
_____
_____
_____
_____
_____
_____

A Framework for Reflection

Gibbs (1998) developed a reflective cycle structure which I have adapted for reflecting on a nursing experience or situation.

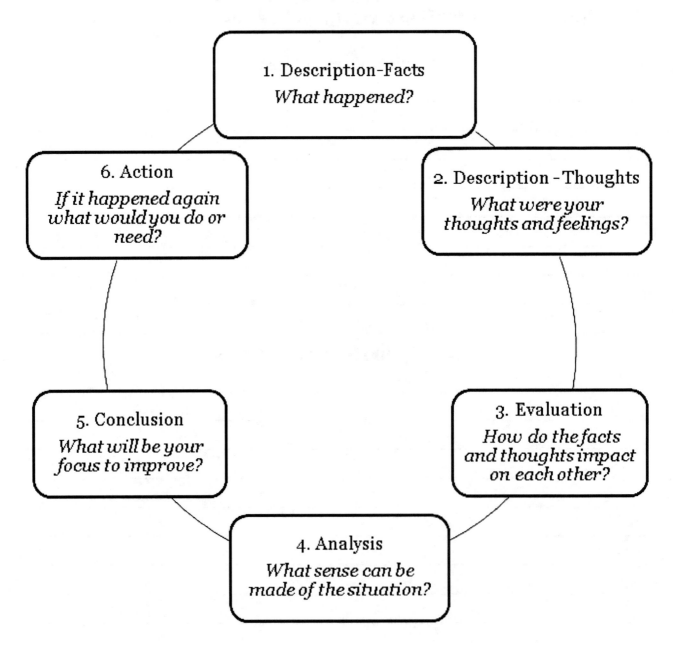

1. Description-Facts
What happened?

2. Description - Thoughts
What were your thoughts and feelings?

3. Evaluation
How do the facts and thoughts impact on each other?

4. Analysis
What sense can be made of the situation?

5. Conclusion
What will be your focus to improve?

6. Action
If it happened again what would you do or need?

Stage 3: Evaluation and Stage 4: Analysis

_____

_____

_____

_____

_____

_____

_____

_____

_____

_____

_____

_____

_____

_____

Stage 5: Conclusions

_____

_____

_____

_____

_____

_____

_____

_____

_____

_____

_____

_____

_____

Relevance to the NMC Code of Practice

Prioritise People ☐   **Practice Effectively** ☐

Preserve Safety ☐   **Promote Professionalism and Trust** ☐

Stage 6: Action Plan For Improvement

_____
_____
_____
_____
_____
_____
_____
_____
_____
_____

Notes and Links to Evidence

_____
_____
_____
_____
_____

Discussed with Professional Assessor ☐

Signature_____**Date Completed**_____

Name_____

NMC Pin Number_____   **Revalidation Due**_____

Incident Date_____   **Date of Reflection**_____

Nature of the CPD activity/practice related feedback

Description Stage 1: Facts

_____
_____
_____
_____
_____
_____
_____
_____
_____
_____

Description Stage 2: Feelings

_____
_____
_____
_____
_____
_____
_____
_____
_____
_____
_____
_____

A Framework for Reflection

Gibbs (1998) developed a reflective cycle structure which I have adapted for reflecting on a nursing experience or situation.

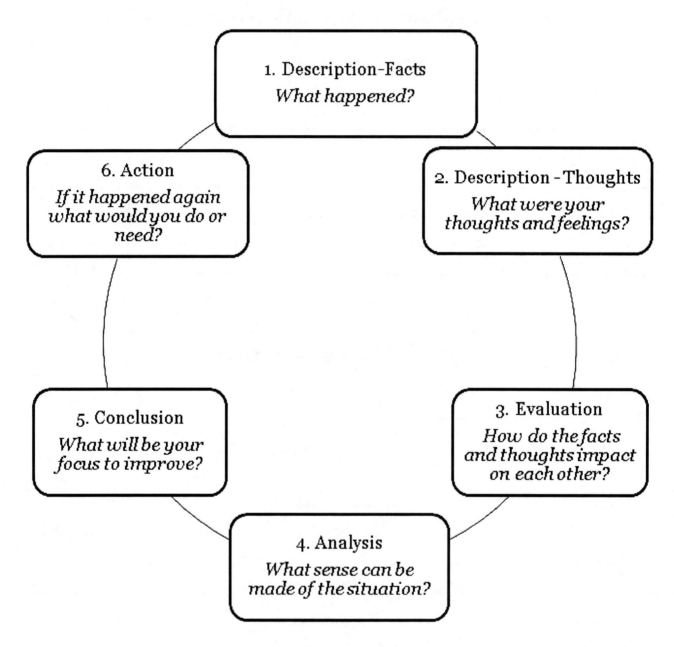

1. Description-Facts
What happened?

2. Description - Thoughts
What were your thoughts and feelings?

3. Evaluation
How do the facts and thoughts impact on each other?

4. Analysis
What sense can be made of the situation?

5. Conclusion
What will be your focus to improve?

6. Action
If it happened again what would you do or need?

Stage 3: Evaluation and Stage 4: Analysis

_____
_____
_____
_____
_____
_____
_____
_____
_____
_____
_____
_____
_____
_____
_____

Stage 5: Conclusions

_____
_____
_____
_____
_____
_____
_____
_____
_____
_____
_____
_____
_____

Relevance to the NMC Code of Practice

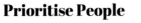

Prioritise People ☐   **Practice Effectively** ☐

Preserve Safety ☐   **Promote Professionalism and Trust** ☐

Stage 6: Action Plan For Improvement

_____
_____
_____
_____
_____
_____
_____
_____
_____
_____

Notes and Links to Evidence

_____
_____
_____
_____
_____

Discussed with Professional Assessor ☐

Signature_____**Date Completed**_____

Name_____

NMC Pin Number_____ **Revalidation Due**_____

Incident Date_____ **Date of Reflection**_____

Nature of the CPD activity/practice related feedback

Description Stage 1: Facts

_____

_____

_____

_____

_____

_____

_____

_____

_____

Description Stage 2: Feelings

_____

_____

_____

_____

_____

_____

_____

_____

_____

_____

A Framework for Reflection

Gibbs (1998) developed a reflective cycle structure which I have adapted for reflecting on a nursing experience or situation.

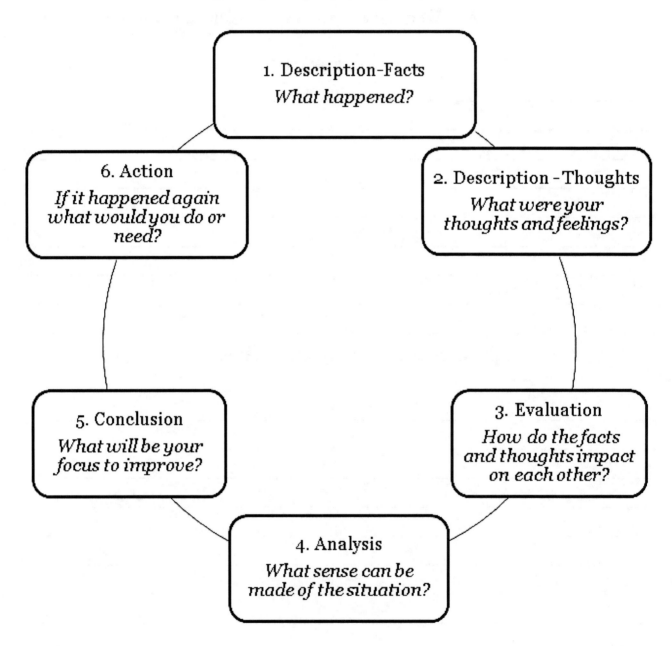

1. Description-Facts
What happened?

2. Description - Thoughts
What were your thoughts and feelings?

3. Evaluation
How do the facts and thoughts impact on each other?

4. Analysis
What sense can be made of the situation?

5. Conclusion
What will be your focus to improve?

6. Action
If it happened again what would you do or need?

Stage 3: Evaluation and Stage 4: Analysis

_____

_____

_____

_____

_____

_____

_____

_____

_____

_____

_____

_____

_____

_____

_____

Stage 5: Conclusions

_____

_____

_____

_____

_____

_____

_____

_____

_____

_____

_____

_____

Relevance to the NMC Code of Practice

Prioritise People ☐ **Practice Effectively** ☐

Preserve Safety ☐ **Promote Professionalism and Trust** ☐

Stage 6: Action Plan For Improvement

_____
_____
_____
_____
_____
_____
_____
_____
_____
_____

Notes and Links to Evidence

_____
_____
_____
_____
_____

Discussed with Professional Assessor ☐

Signature_____**Date Completed**_____

Name_____

NMC Pin Number_____ **Revalidation Due**_____

Incident Date_____ **Date of Reflection**_____

Nature of the CPD activity/practice related feedback

Description Stage 1: Facts

_____
_____
_____
_____
_____
_____
_____
_____
_____

Description Stage 2: Feelings

_____
_____
_____
_____
_____
_____
_____
_____
_____

A Framework for Reflection

Gibbs (1998) developed a reflective cycle structure which I have adapted for reflecting on a nursing experience or situation.

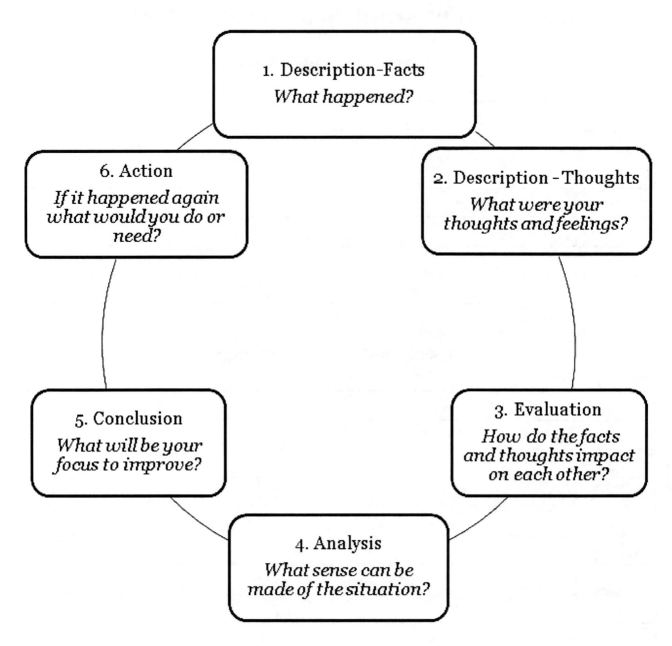

1. Description-Facts
What happened?

2. Description - Thoughts
What were your thoughts and feelings?

3. Evaluation
How do the facts and thoughts impact on each other?

4. Analysis
What sense can be made of the situation?

5. Conclusion
What will be your focus to improve?

6. Action
If it happened again what would you do or need?

Stage 3: Evaluation and Stage 4: Analysis

_____
_____
_____
_____
_____
_____
_____
_____
_____
_____
_____
_____
_____
_____
_____
_____

Stage 5: Conclusions

_____
_____
_____
_____
_____
_____
_____
_____
_____
_____
_____
_____
_____

Relevance to the NMC Code of Practice

Prioritise People ☐   **Practice Effectively** ☐

Preserve Safety ☐   **Promote Professionalism and Trust** ☐

Stage 6: Action Plan For Improvement

_____

_____

_____

_____

_____

_____

_____

_____

_____

_____

Notes and Links to Evidence

_____

_____

_____

_____

_____

Discussed with Professional Assessor ☐

Signature_____**Date Completed**_____

Name_____

NMC Pin Number_____   **Revalidation Due**_____

Incident Date_____   **Date of Reflection**_____

Nature of the CPD activity/practice related feedback

Description Stage 1: Facts

_____
_____
_____
_____
_____
_____
_____
_____
_____

Description Stage 2: Feelings

_____
_____
_____
_____
_____
_____
_____
_____
_____
_____

A Framework for Reflection

Gibbs (1998) developed a reflective cycle structure which I have adapted for reflecting on a nursing experience or situation.

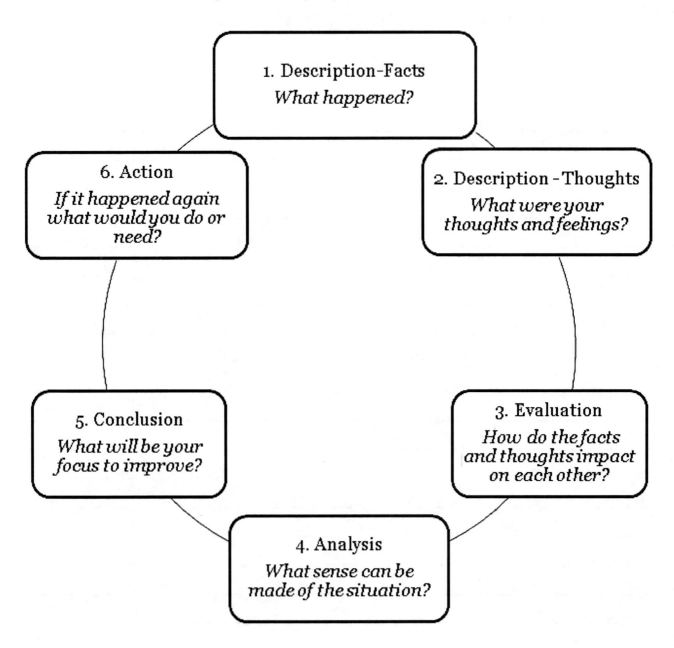

1. Description-Facts
What happened?

2. Description -Thoughts
What were your thoughts and feelings?

3. Evaluation
How do the facts and thoughts impact on each other?

4. Analysis
What sense can be made of the situation?

5. Conclusion
What will be your focus to improve?

6. Action
If it happened again what would you do or need?

Stage 3: Evaluation and Stage 4: Analysis

_____
_____
_____
_____
_____
_____
_____
_____
_____
_____
_____
_____
_____
_____
_____
_____
_____

Stage 5: Conclusions

_____
_____
_____
_____
_____
_____
_____
_____
_____
_____
_____
_____
_____
_____
_____

Relevance to the NMC Code of Practice

Prioritise People ☐   **Practice Effectively** ☐

Preserve Safety ☐   **Promote Professionalism and Trust** ☐

Stage 6: Action Plan For Improvement

_____
_____
_____
_____
_____
_____
_____
_____
_____

Notes and Links to Evidence

_____
_____
_____
_____
_____

Discussed with Professional Assessor ☐

Signature_____**Date Completed**_____

Name_____

NMC Pin Number_____   **Revalidation Due**_____

Incident Date_____   **Date of Reflection**_____

Nature of the CPD activity/practice related feedback

Description Stage 1: Facts

_____

_____

_____

_____

_____

_____

_____

_____

Description Stage 2: Feelings

_____

_____

_____

_____

_____

_____

_____

_____

_____

_____

A Framework for Reflection

Gibbs (1998) developed a reflective cycle structure which I have adapted for reflecting on a nursing experience or situation.

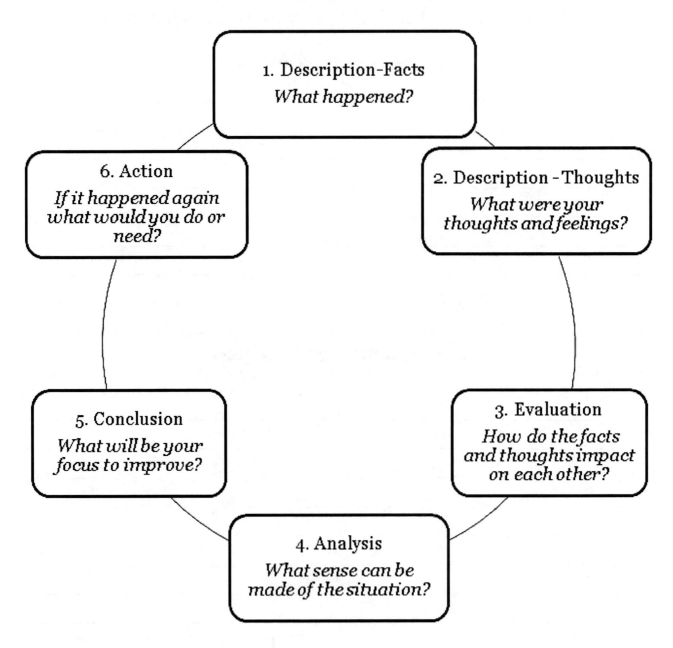

1. Description-Facts
   What happened?

2. Description - Thoughts
   What were your thoughts and feelings?

3. Evaluation
   How do the facts and thoughts impact on each other?

4. Analysis
   What sense can be made of the situation?

5. Conclusion
   What will be your focus to improve?

6. Action
   If it happened again what would you do or need?

Stage 3: Evaluation and Stage 4: Analysis

_____

_____

_____

_____

_____

_____

_____

_____

_____

_____

_____

_____

_____

_____

_____

_____

_____

Stage 5: Conclusions

_____

_____

_____

_____

_____

_____

_____

_____

_____

_____

_____

_____

_____

_____

_____

Relevance to the NMC Code of Practice

Prioritise People ☐   **Practice Effectively** ☐

Preserve Safety ☐   **Promote Professionalism and Trust** ☐

Stage 6: Action Plan For Improvement

_____
_____
_____
_____
_____
_____
_____
_____
_____
_____

Notes and Links to Evidence

_____
_____
_____
_____
_____

Discussed with Professional Assessor ☐

Signature_____**Date Completed**_____

Name_____

NMC Pin Number_____ **Revalidation Due**_____

Incident Date_____ **Date of Reflection**_____

Nature of the CPD activity/practice related feedback

Description Stage 1: Facts

_____

_____

_____

_____

_____

_____

_____

_____

Description Stage 2: Feelings

_____

_____

_____

_____

_____

_____

_____

_____

A Framework for Reflection

Gibbs (1998) developed a reflective cycle structure which I have adapted for reflecting on a nursing experience or situation.

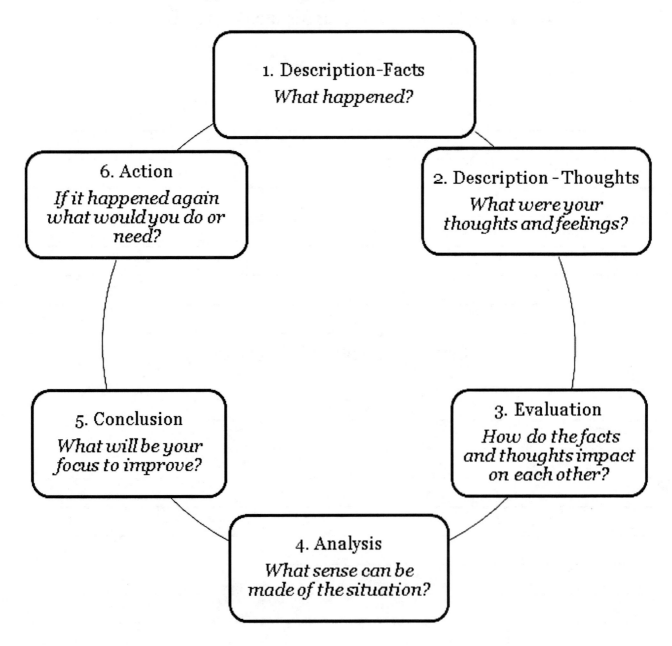

1. Description-Facts
What happened?

2. Description - Thoughts
What were your thoughts and feelings?

3. Evaluation
How do the facts and thoughts impact on each other?

4. Analysis
What sense can be made of the situation?

5. Conclusion
What will be your focus to improve?

6. Action
If it happened again what would you do or need?

Stage 3: Evaluation and Stage 4: Analysis

Stage 5: Conclusions

Relevance to the NMC Code of Practice

Prioritise People ☐   **Practice Effectively** ☐

Preserve Safety ☐   **Promote Professionalism and Trust** ☐

Stage 6: Action Plan For Improvement

_____

_____

_____

_____

_____

_____

_____

_____

_____

_____

Notes and Links to Evidence

_____

_____

_____

_____

_____

Discussed with Professional Assessor ☐

Signature_____**Date Completed**_____

Name_____

NMC Pin Number_____ **Revalidation Due**_____

Incident Date_____ **Date of Reflection**_____

Nature of the CPD activity/practice related feedback

Description Stage 1: Facts

_____
_____
_____
_____
_____
_____
_____
_____
_____

Description Stage 2: Feelings

_____
_____
_____
_____
_____
_____
_____
_____
_____
_____
_____

A Framework for Reflection

Gibbs (1998) developed a reflective cycle structure which I have adapted for reflecting on a nursing experience or situation.

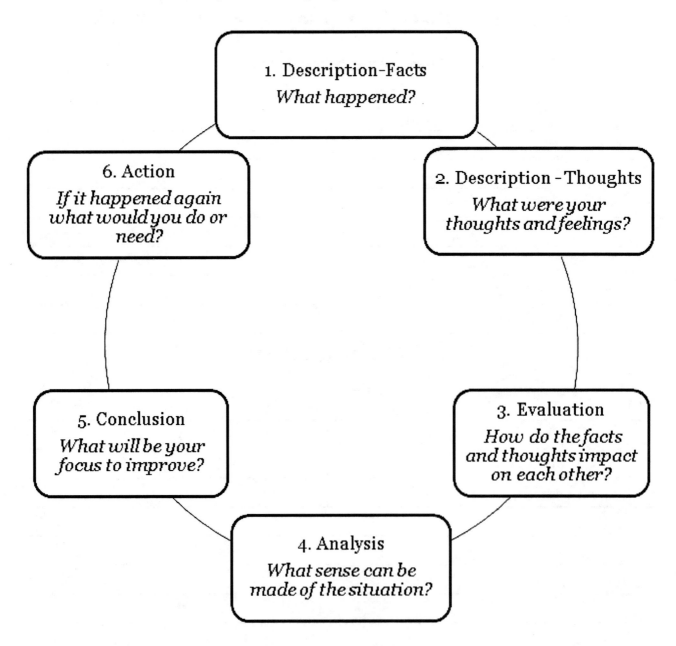

1. Description-Facts
What happened?

2. Description - Thoughts
What were your thoughts and feelings?

3. Evaluation
How do the facts and thoughts impact on each other?

4. Analysis
What sense can be made of the situation?

5. Conclusion
What will be your focus to improve?

6. Action
If it happened again what would you do or need?

Stage 3: Evaluation and Stage 4: Analysis

_____
_____
_____
_____
_____
_____
_____
_____
_____
_____
_____
_____
_____
_____
_____
_____
_____

Stage 5: Conclusions

_____
_____
_____
_____
_____
_____
_____
_____
_____
_____
_____
_____
_____
_____

Relevance to the NMC Code of Practice

Prioritise People ☐   **Practice Effectively** ☐

Preserve Safety ☐   **Promote Professionalism and Trust** ☐

Stage 6: Action Plan For Improvement

_____
_____
_____
_____
_____
_____
_____
_____
_____
_____

Notes and Links to Evidence

_____
_____
_____
_____
_____

Discussed with Professional Assessor ☐

Signature_____**Date Completed**_____

Name_____

NMC Pin Number_____ **Revalidation Due**_____

Incident Date_____ **Date of Reflection**_____

Nature of the CPD activity/practice related feedback

Description Stage 1: Facts

_____
_____
_____
_____
_____
_____
_____
_____
_____

Description Stage 2: Feelings

_____
_____
_____
_____
_____
_____
_____
_____
_____
_____

A Framework for Reflection

Gibbs (1998) developed a reflective cycle structure which I have adapted for reflecting on a nursing experience or situation.

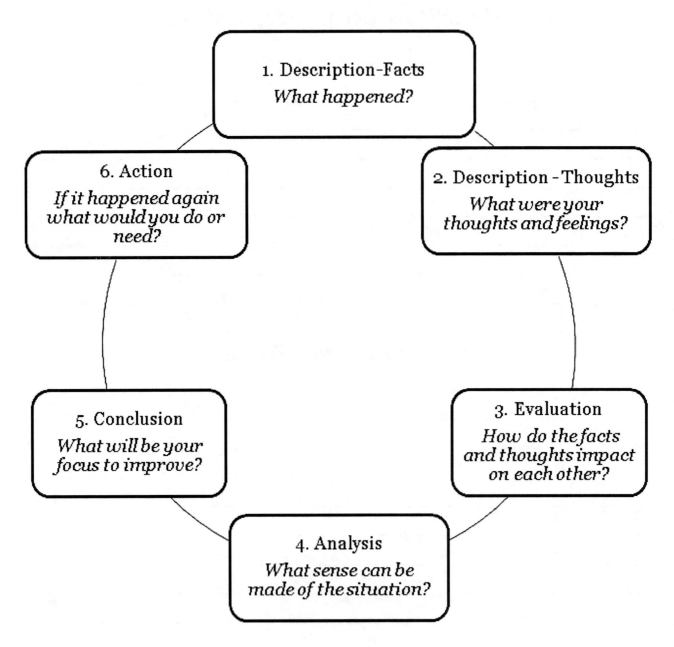

Stage 3: Evaluation and Stage 4: Analysis

_____
_____
_____
_____
_____
_____
_____
_____
_____
_____
_____
_____
_____
_____
_____
_____
_____

Stage 5: Conclusions

_____
_____
_____
_____
_____
_____
_____
_____
_____
_____
_____
_____
_____
_____

Relevance to the NMC Code of Practice

Prioritise People ☐   **Practice Effectively** ☐

Preserve Safety ☐   **Promote Professionalism and Trust** ☐

Stage 6: Action Plan For Improvement

_____
_____
_____
_____
_____
_____
_____
_____
_____
_____

Notes and Links to Evidence

_____
_____
_____
_____
_____

Discussed with Professional Assessor ☐

Signature_____**Date Completed**_____

Name_____

NMC Pin Number_____ **Revalidation Due**_____

Incident Date_____ **Date of Reflection**_____

Nature of the CPD activity/practice related feedback

Description Stage 1: Facts

_____
_____
_____
_____
_____
_____
_____
_____
_____

Description Stage 2: Feelings

_____
_____
_____
_____
_____
_____
_____
_____
_____
_____

A Framework for Reflection

Gibbs (1998) developed a reflective cycle structure which I have adapted for reflecting on a nursing experience or situation.

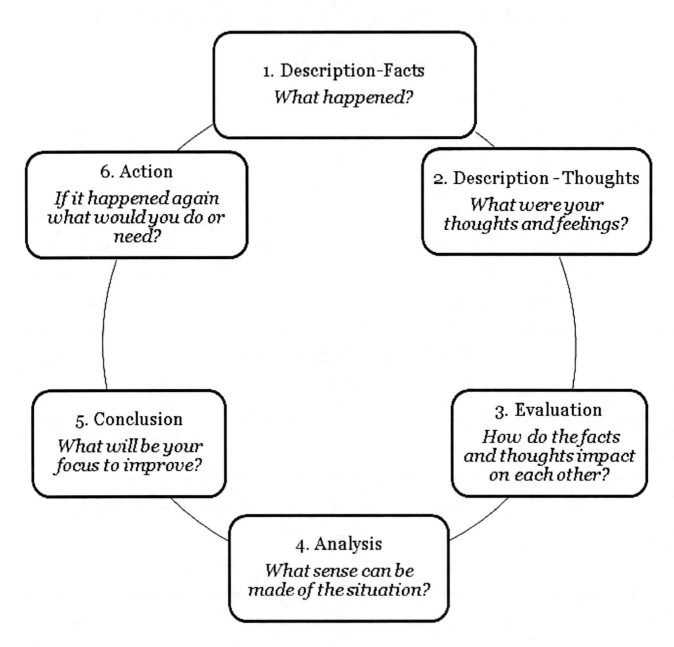

1. Description-Facts
What happened?

6. Action
If it happened again what would you do or need?

2. Description - Thoughts
What were your thoughts and feelings?

5. Conclusion
What will be your focus to improve?

3. Evaluation
How do the facts and thoughts impact on each other?

4. Analysis
What sense can be made of the situation?

Stage 3: Evaluation and Stage 4: Analysis

_____
_____
_____
_____
_____
_____
_____
_____
_____
_____
_____
_____
_____
_____
_____
_____

Stage 5: Conclusions

_____
_____
_____
_____
_____
_____
_____
_____
_____
_____
_____
_____
_____

Relevance to the NMC Code of Practice

Prioritise People ☐   **Practice Effectively** ☐

Preserve Safety ☐   **Promote Professionalism and Trust** ☐

Stage 6: Action Plan For Improvement

_____
_____
_____
_____
_____
_____
_____
_____
_____
_____

Notes and Links to Evidence

_____
_____
_____
_____
_____

Discussed with Professional Assessor ☐

Signature_____**Date Completed**_____

Name_____

NMC Pin Number_____   **Revalidation Due**_____

Incident Date_____   **Date of Reflection**_____

Nature of the CPD activity/practice related feedback

Description Stage 1: Facts

_____
_____
_____
_____
_____
_____
_____
_____
_____

Description Stage 2: Feelings

_____
_____
_____
_____
_____
_____
_____
_____
_____
_____
_____

A Framework for Reflection

Gibbs (1998) developed a reflective cycle structure which I have adapted for reflecting on a nursing experience or situation.

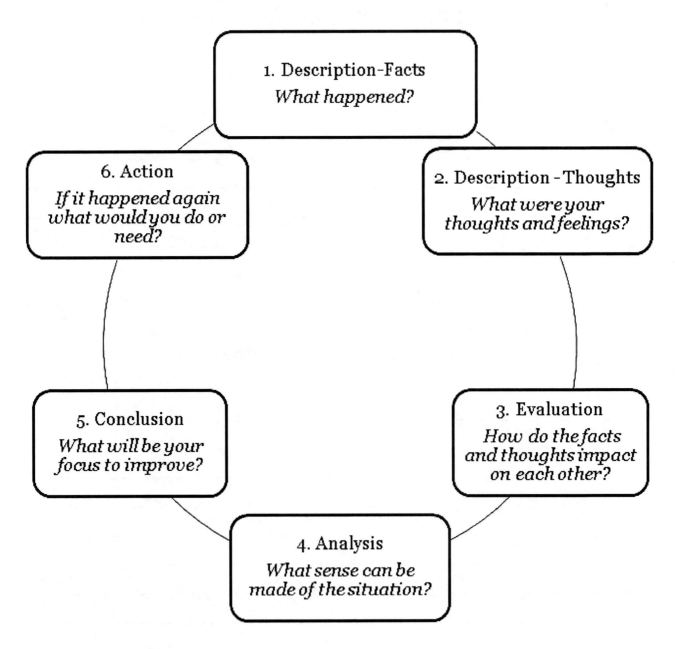

1. Description-Facts
What happened?

2. Description - Thoughts
What were your thoughts and feelings?

3. Evaluation
How do the facts and thoughts impact on each other?

4. Analysis
What sense can be made of the situation?

5. Conclusion
What will be your focus to improve?

6. Action
If it happened again what would you do or need?

Stage 3: Evaluation and Stage 4: Analysis

_____

_____

_____

_____

_____

_____

_____

_____

_____

_____

_____

_____

_____

_____

_____

_____

Stage 5: Conclusions

_____

_____

_____

_____

_____

_____

_____

_____

_____

_____

_____

_____

_____

_____

Relevance to the NMC Code of Practice

Prioritise People ☐   **Practice Effectively** ☐

Preserve Safety ☐   **Promote Professionalism and Trust** ☐

Stage 6: Action Plan For Improvement

_____
_____
_____
_____
_____
_____
_____
_____
_____
_____

Notes and Links to Evidence

_____
_____
_____
_____
_____

Discussed with Professional Assessor ☐

Signature_____**Date Completed**_____

Name_____

NMC Pin Number_____   Revalidation Due_____

Incident Date_____   Date of Reflection_____

Nature of the CPD activity/practice related feedback

Description Stage 1: Facts

_____

_____

_____

_____

_____

_____

_____

_____

_____

Description Stage 2: Feelings

_____

_____

_____

_____

_____

_____

_____

_____

_____

A Framework for Reflection

Gibbs (1998) developed a reflective cycle structure which I have adapted for reflecting on a nursing experience or situation.

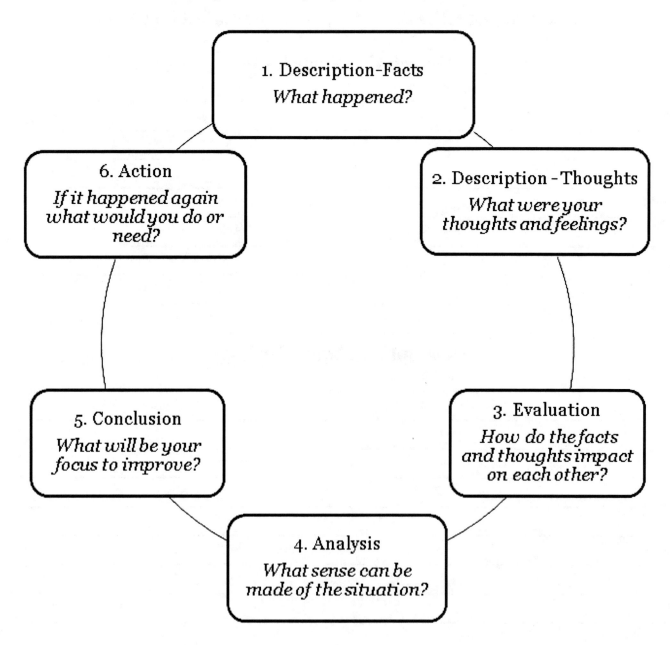

1. Description-Facts
What happened?

2. Description - Thoughts
What were your thoughts and feelings?

3. Evaluation
How do the facts and thoughts impact on each other?

4. Analysis
What sense can be made of the situation?

5. Conclusion
What will be your focus to improve?

6. Action
If it happened again what would you do or need?

Stage 3: Evaluation and Stage 4: Analysis

_____
_____
_____
_____
_____
_____
_____
_____
_____
_____
_____
_____
_____
_____
_____

Stage 5: Conclusions

_____
_____
_____
_____
_____
_____
_____
_____
_____
_____
_____
_____
_____

Relevance to the NMC Code of Practice

Prioritise People ☐

Practice Effectively ☐

Preserve Safety ☐

Promote Professionalism and Trust ☐

Stage 6: Action Plan For Improvement

_____
_____
_____
_____
_____
_____
_____
_____
_____
_____

Notes and Links to Evidence

_____
_____
_____
_____
_____

Discussed with Professional Assessor ☐

Signature_____**Date Completed**_____

Name_____

NMC Pin Number_____   **Revalidation Due**_____

Incident Date_____   **Date of Reflection**_____

Nature of the CPD activity/practice related feedback

Description Stage 1: Facts

_____
_____
_____
_____
_____
_____
_____
_____
_____

Description Stage 2: Feelings

_____
_____
_____
_____
_____
_____
_____
_____
_____

A Framework for Reflection

Gibbs (1998) developed a reflective cycle structure which I have adapted for reflecting on a nursing experience or situation.

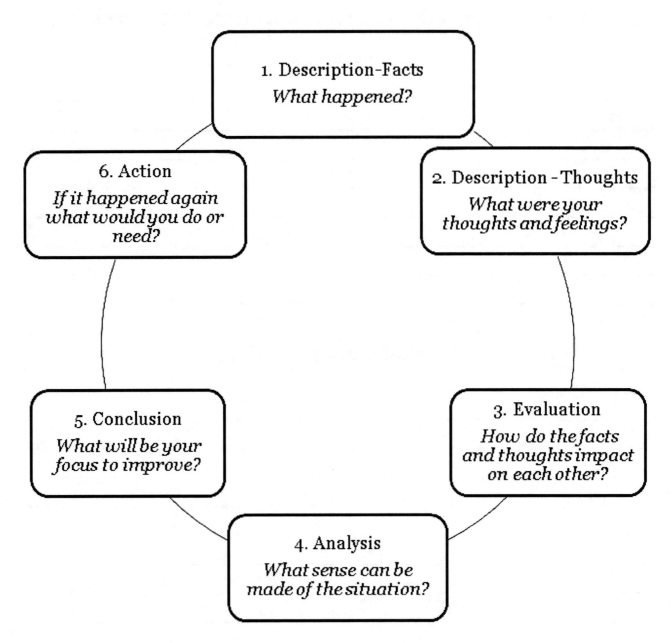

Stage 3: Evaluation and Stage 4: Analysis

_____
_____
_____
_____
_____
_____
_____
_____
_____
_____
_____
_____
_____
_____
_____

Stage 5: Conclusions

_____
_____
_____
_____
_____
_____
_____
_____
_____
_____
_____
_____
_____
_____

Relevance to the NMC Code of Practice

Prioritise People ☐   **Practice Effectively** ☐

Preserve Safety ☐   **Promote Professionalism and Trust** ☐

Stage 6: Action Plan For Improvement

_____
_____
_____
_____
_____
_____
_____
_____
_____
_____

Notes and Links to Evidence

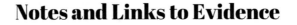

_____
_____
_____
_____
_____

Discussed with Professional Assessor ☐

Signature_____ **Date Completed**_____

Name_____

NMC Pin Number_____ **Revalidation Due**_____

Incident Date_____ **Date of Reflection**_____

Nature of the CPD activity/practice related feedback

Description Stage 1: Facts

_____
_____
_____
_____
_____
_____
_____
_____
_____

Description Stage 2: Feelings

_____
_____
_____
_____
_____
_____
_____
_____
_____
_____

A Framework for Reflection

Gibbs (1998) developed a reflective cycle structure which I have adapted for reflecting on a nursing experience or situation.

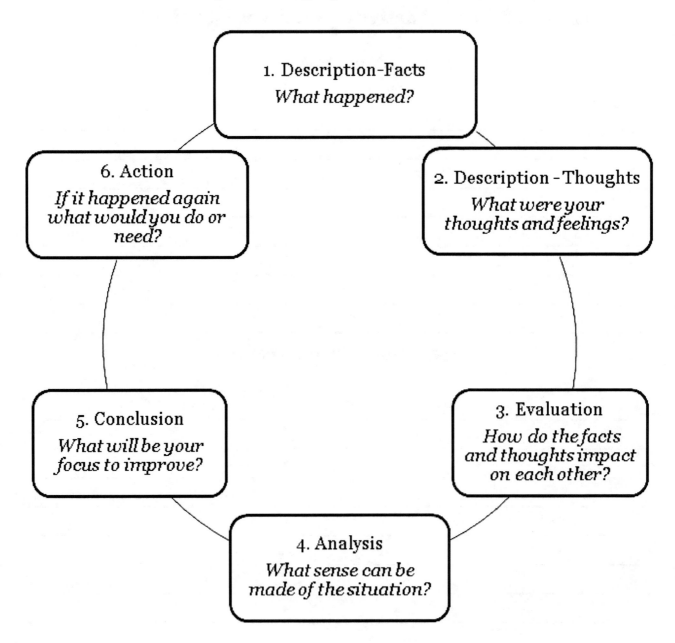

1. Description-Facts
What happened?

2. Description - Thoughts
What were your thoughts and feelings?

3. Evaluation
How do the facts and thoughts impact on each other?

4. Analysis
What sense can be made of the situation?

5. Conclusion
What will be your focus to improve?

6. Action
If it happened again what would you do or need?

Stage 3: Evaluation and Stage 4: Analysis

_____

_____

_____

_____

_____

_____

_____

_____

_____

_____

_____

_____

_____

Stage 5: Conclusions

_____

_____

_____

_____

_____

_____

_____

_____

_____

_____

_____

_____

Relevance to the NMC Code of Practice

Prioritise People ☐   **Practice Effectively** ☐

Preserve Safety ☐   **Promote Professionalism and Trust** ☐

Stage 6: Action Plan For Improvement

_____
_____
_____
_____
_____
_____
_____
_____
_____

Notes and Links to Evidence

_____
_____
_____
_____
_____

Discussed with Professional Assessor ☐

Signature_____**Date Completed**_____

Name_____

NMC Pin Number_____   **Revalidation Due**_____

Incident Date_____   **Date of Reflection**_____

Nature of the CPD activity/practice related feedback

Description Stage 1: Facts

_____

_____

_____

_____

_____

_____

_____

_____

_____

Description Stage 2: Feelings

_____

_____

_____

_____

_____

_____

_____

_____

_____

A Framework for Reflection

Gibbs (1998) developed a reflective cycle structure which I have adapted for reflecting on a nursing experience or situation.

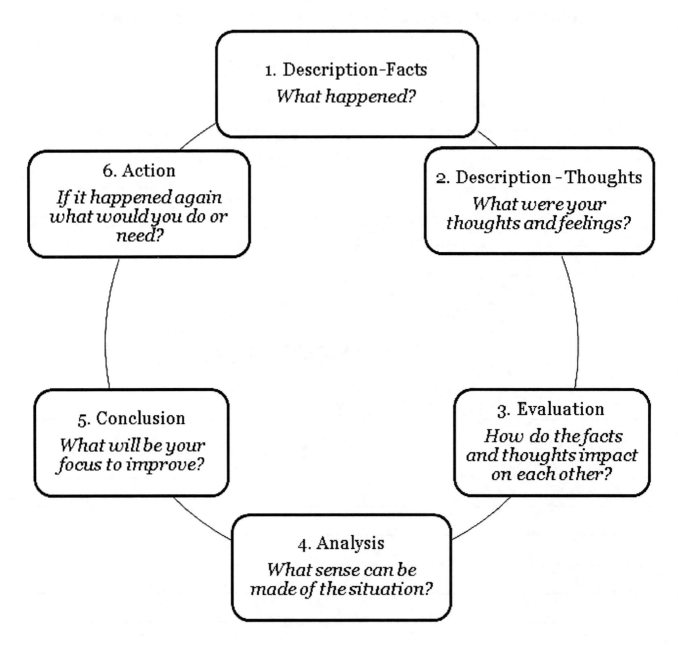

1. Description-Facts
What happened?

2. Description -Thoughts
What were your thoughts and feelings?

3. Evaluation
How do the facts and thoughts impact on each other?

4. Analysis
What sense can be made of the situation?

5. Conclusion
What will be your focus to improve?

6. Action
If it happened again what would you do or need?

Stage 3: Evaluation and Stage 4: Analysis

_____

_____

_____

_____

_____

_____

_____

_____

_____

_____

_____

_____

_____

_____

_____

_____

_____

Stage 5: Conclusions

_____

_____

_____

_____

_____

_____

_____

_____

_____

_____

_____

_____

_____

_____

Relevance to the NMC Code of Practice

Prioritise People ☐ **Practice Effectively** ☐

Preserve Safety ☐ **Promote Professionalism and Trust** ☐

Stage 6: Action Plan For Improvement

_____
_____
_____
_____
_____
_____
_____
_____
_____
_____

Notes and Links to Evidence

_____
_____
_____
_____
_____

Discussed with Professional Assessor ☐

Signature_____**Date Completed**_____

Name_____

NMC Pin Number_____   Revalidation Due_____

Incident Date_____   Date of Reflection_____

Nature of the CPD activity/practice related feedback

Description Stage 1: Facts

_____

_____

_____

_____

_____

_____

_____

_____

_____

Description Stage 2: Feelings

_____

_____

_____

_____

_____

_____

_____

_____

_____

_____

_____

A Framework for Reflection

Gibbs (1998) developed a reflective cycle structure which I have adapted for reflecting on a nursing experience or situation.

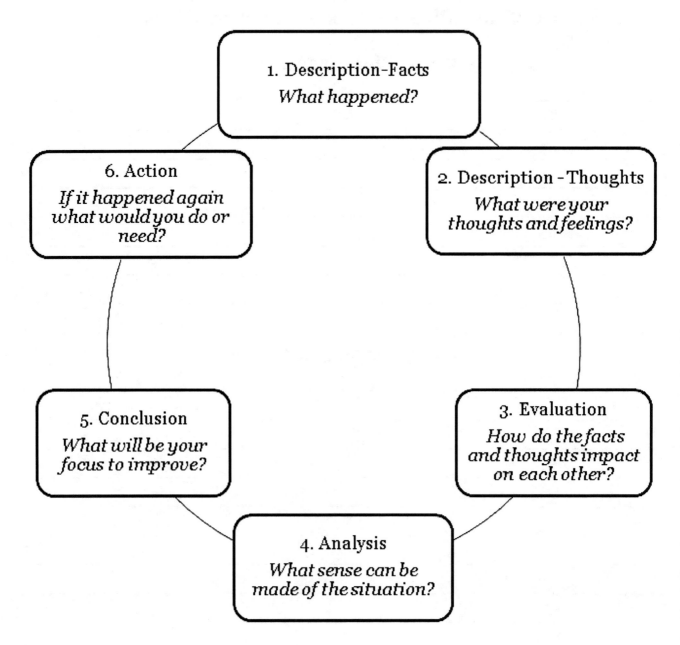

1. Description-Facts

What happened?

2. Description - Thoughts

What were your thoughts and feelings?

3. Evaluation

How do the facts and thoughts impact on each other?

4. Analysis

What sense can be made of the situation?

5. Conclusion

What will be your focus to improve?

6. Action

If it happened again what would you do or need?

Stage 3: Evaluation and Stage 4: Analysis

_____

_____

_____

_____

_____

_____

_____

_____

_____

_____

_____

_____

_____

_____

_____

_____

Stage 5: Conclusions

_____

_____

_____

_____

_____

_____

_____

_____

_____

_____

_____

_____

_____

Relevance to the NMC Code of Practice

Prioritise People ☐   **Practice Effectively** ☐

Preserve Safety ☐   **Promote Professionalism and Trust** ☐

Stage 6: Action Plan For Improvement

_____
_____
_____
_____
_____
_____
_____
_____
_____
_____

Notes and Links to Evidence

_____
_____
_____
_____
_____

Discussed with Professional Assessor ☐

Signature_____**Date Completed**_____

Professional Development Assessor

Name of Assessor_____

NMC Pin Number_____ **Date**_____

Email Address _____

Professional Address _____

_____

_____

Registrant Name _____

NMC Pin
Number_____ **Date**_____

Number of Reflections Discussed_____

I confirm that I have discussed the number of reflective accounts listed above, with the named registrant, as part of the professional development discussion and in line with guidance from the Nursing Midwifery Council

Signature _____

Professional Development Assessor

Name of Assessor_____

NMC Pin Number_____ **Date**_____

Email Address _____

Professional Address _____

_____

_____

Registrant Name _____

NMC Pin
Number_____ **Date**_____

Number of Reflections Discussed_____

I confirm that I have discussed the number of reflective accounts listed above, with the named registrant, as part of the professional development discussion and in line with guidance from the Nursing Midwifery Council

Signature _____

Professional Development Assessor

Name of Assessor_____

NMC Pin Number_____ **Date**_____

Email Address _____

Professional Address _____

_____

_____

Registrant Name _____

NMC Pin
Number_____ **Date**_____

Number of Reflections Discussed_____

I confirm that I have discussed the number of reflective accounts listed above, with the named registrant, as part of the professional development discussion and in line with guidance from the Nursing Midwifery Council

Signature _____

Professional Development Assessor

Name of Assessor_____

NMC Pin Number_____ **Date**_____

Email Address _____

Professional Address _____

_____

_____

Registrant Name _____

NMC Pin
Number_____   **Date**_____

Number of Reflections Discussed_____

I confirm that I have discussed the number of reflective accounts listed above, with the named registrant, as part of the professional development discussion and in line with guidance from the Nursing Midwifery Council

Signature _____

Professional Development Assessor

Name of Assessor_____

NMC Pin Number_____ **Date**_____

Email Address _____

Professional Address _____

_____

_____

Registrant Name _____

NMC Pin
Number_____   **Date**_____

Number of Reflections Discussed_____

I confirm that I have discussed the number of reflective accounts listed above, with the named registrant, as part of the professional development discussion and in line with guidance from the Nursing Midwifery Council

Signature _____

Professional Development Assessor

Name of Assessor_____

NMC Pin Number_____ **Date**_____

Email Address _____

Professional Address _____

_____

_____

Registrant Name _____

NMC Pin

Number_____   **Date**_____

Number of Reflections Discussed_____

I confirm that I have discussed the number of reflective accounts listed above, with the named registrant, as part of the professional development discussion and in line with guidance from the Nursing Midwifery Council

Signature _____

Professional Development Assessor

Name of Assessor_____

NMC Pin Number_____ **Date**_____

Email Address _____

Professional Address _____

_____

_____

Registrant Name _____

NMC Pin
Number_____ **Date**_____

Number of Reflections Discussed_____

I confirm that I have discussed the number of reflective accounts listed above, with the named registrant, as part of the professional development discussion and in line with guidance from the Nursing Midwifery Council

Signature _____

Professional Development Assessor

Name of Assessor _____

NMC Pin Number _____ **Date** _____

Email Address _____

Professional Address _____

_____

_____

Registrant Name _____

NMC Pin
Number _____ **Date** _____

Number of Reflections Discussed _____

I confirm that I have discussed the number of reflective accounts listed above, with the named registrant, as part of the professional development discussion and in line with guidance from the Nursing Midwifery Council

Signature _____

Professional Development Assessor

Name of Assessor_____

NMC Pin Number_____ **Date**_____

Email Address _____

Professional Address _____

_____

_____

Registrant Name _____

NMC Pin
Number_____ **Date**_____

Number of Reflections Discussed_____

I confirm that I have discussed the number of reflective accounts listed above, with the named registrant, as part of the professional development discussion and in line with guidance from the Nursing Midwifery Council

Signature _____

Professional Development Assessor

Name of Assessor_____

NMC Pin Number_____ **Date**_____

Email Address _____

Professional Address _____

_____

_____

Registrant Name _____

**NMC Pin
Number**_____   **Date**_____

Number of Reflections Discussed_____

I confirm that I have discussed the number of reflective accounts listed above, with the named registrant, as part of the professional development discussion and in line with guidance from the Nursing Midwifery Council

Signature _____

Professional Development Assessor

Name of Assessor_____

NMC Pin Number_____ **Date**_____

Email Address _____

Professional Address _____

_____

_____

Registrant Name _____

NMC Pin

Number_____ **Date**_____

Number of Reflections Discussed_____

I confirm that I have discussed the number of reflective accounts listed above, with the named registrant, as part of the professional development discussion and in line with guidance from the Nursing Midwifery Council

Signature _____

Professional Development Assessor

Name of Assessor_____

NMC Pin Number_____ **Date**_____

Email Address _____

Professional Address _____

_____

_____

Registrant Name _____

NMC Pin
Number_____ **Date**_____

Number of Reflections Discussed_____

I confirm that I have discussed the number of reflective accounts listed above, with the named registrant, as part of the professional development discussion and in line with guidance from the Nursing Midwifery Council

Signature _____

Before You Go

I hope you have found this reflection diary useful? If so, I would appreciate an honest review on the website where you bought it.

Also, if you have any comments on how I can improve this book then I would love to hear from you.

This is revision number 2 after a few such suggestions.

Contact me at: jane.coombs@workingwellsolutions.com or via my website at www.workingwellsolutions.com.

My mission:

Influencing and advocating ethical health and safety practice on every level, making it accessible and welcoming for those most in need.

Jane Coombs January 2016

Other Books By Me

"How to Look After the Elf in Health and Safety"
For safety professionals and manager's – how to put health in the risk
assessment process in your workplace

"The Good, the Bad, and the Smugly:
Behind the Scenes at Occupational Health"
Interesting and challenging health situations
at work from my perspective

"How to Start a Healthy Business:
An Insider's Guide to Occupational Health Success"
Starting you own health business and aiming at workplaces?
This book is for you.

"The Manager's Ultimate Guide to
Health and Wellbeing at Work
Answers and Help You Need"
References and answers to the most asked questions
in occupational health from Managers and Human Resources professionals